THE ULTIMATE DIVERTICULITIS COOKBOOK

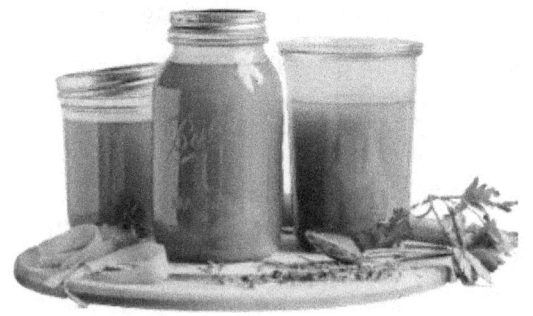

Gluten-Free Anti Inflammatory Recipes for Digestive Health

Linda Carlucci

Copyright © 2024 by Linda Carlucci

All rights reserved. No part of this book may be reproduced, stored, or transmitted by any means whether auditory, graphic, mechanical, or electronic without written permission of the author, except in the case of brief excerpts used in critical articles and reviews.

All the people depicted in stock imagery are models, and such images are being used for illustrative purposes only.

DISCLAIMER

This cookbook is intended to provide general information and recipes.

The recipes provided in this cookbook are not intended to replace or be a substitute for medical advice from a physician.

The reader should consult a healthcare professional for any specific medical advice, diagnosis or treatment.

Any specific dietary advice provided in this cookbook is not intended to replace or be a substitute for medical advice from a physician.

The author is not responsible or liable for any adverse effects experienced by readers of this cookbook as a result of following the recipes or dietary advice provided.

The author makes no representations or warranties of any kind (express or implied) as to the accuracy, completeness, reliability or suitability of the recipes provided in this cookbook.

The author disclaims any and all liability for any damages arising out of the use or misuse of the recipes provided in this cookbook. The reader must also take care to ensure that the recipes provided in this cookbook are prepared and cooked safely.

The recipes provided in this cookbook are for informational purposes only and should not be used as a substitute for professional medical advice, diagnosis or treatment.

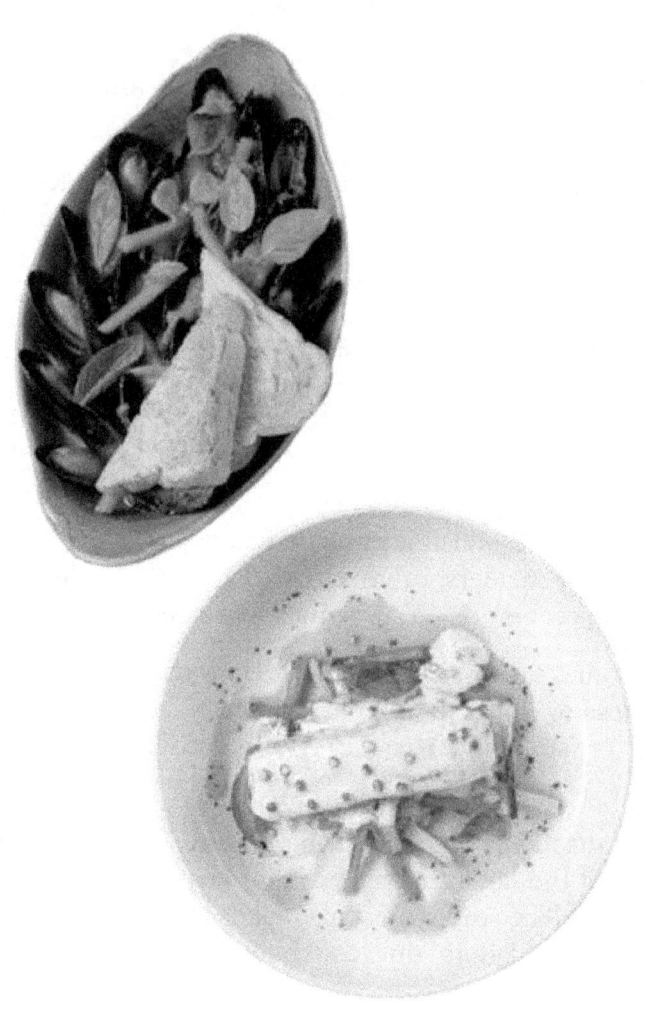

TABLE OF CONTENTS

INTRODUCTION 11

CHAPTER 1 13

    6 COMMON RISK FACTORS THAT LEAD TO THE DEVELOPMENT OF DIVERTICULITIS 13

    SIMPLE STRATEGIES FOR RELIEVING SYMPTOMS 15

    FOODS TO AVOID FOR DIVERTICULITIS PATIENTS............. 18

    THE 3 SYMPTOM-SPECIFIC STEPS DIET 21

CHAPTER 2 25

    NUTRITIOUS RECIPES FOR A DIVERTICULITIS DIET 25

    CLEAR LIQUID DIET FOR FLARE UPS 25

    BREAKFAST 25

    Vegetable Broth... 25

    Clear Herbal Tea 26

    Coconut Water... 27

    Clear Sports Drink 28

    Blueberry, Spinach and Banana Smoothie 29

    Apple Flavored Popsicles.. 30

    Clear Protein Drink 31

    LUNCH.. 32

    Chicken Broth 32

Clear Vegetable Soup 33

Clear Fish Broth 35

Apple Juice 36

Beef Soup 37

Gelatin Desserts 38

Apple, Pear, and Carrot Smoothie 39

DINNER 40

Clear Beef Broth 40

Clear Miso Soup 42

Clear Chicken Noodle Soup (Strained) 43

Fruit Juice Gelatin 45

Clear Chicken Soup 46

White Grape Juice 48

Clear Strained Fruit Juice 48

LOW FIBER DIET 50

BREAKFAST 50

Refined Oatmeal with Sliced Strawberries 50

Cucumber Smoothie with Plain Yogurt 51

Egg White Omelet with Cooked Carrots 52

Plain Yogurt with Mashed Ripe Banana 53

Scrambled Eggs with Well-Cooked Spinach 54

White Toast with Creamy Peanut Butter 55

Poached Eggs on White Toast with Peeled and Cooked Tomatoes . 56

Rice Cakes with Cream Cheese and Sliced Avocado 58

LUNCH 59

Chicken and Rice Soup 59

Mashed Potatoes with Grilled Chicken Breast 60

Tuna Salad on White Bread 61

Scrambled Eggs with Soft-Cooked Vegetables 63

Baked Salmon with Steamed Carrots and White Rice 64

Turkey and Cheese Sandwich on White Bread 65

Vegetable Broth with Soft-Cooked Noodles 67

Salmon Vegetable Soup 68

Plain Pasta with Butter or Olive Oil 69

DINNER 71

Baked Cod with Quinoa Pilaf and Steamed Green Beans 71

Turkey Chili Made with Ground Turkey, Tomatoes, and Kidney Beans 73

Roast Chicken with Roasted Sweet Potatoes and Steamed Broccoli 75

Beef Stew Made with Tender Beef, Potatoes, and Well-Cooked Carrots 76

Egg Drop Soup with Cooked Chicken and Soft Tofu 78

Vegetable Stir-Fry with Tofu and White Rice 80

Baked Chicken Breast with Mashed Potatoes and Steamed Carrots 81

Poached Salmon with White Rice and Cooked Spinach 83

HIGH FIBER DIET 84

BREAKFAST 84

Whole Grain Toast with Avocado and Poached Eggs 84

Greek Yogurt Parfait with Berries and Granola 86

Whole Grain Pancakes Topped with Greek Yogurt and Mixed Berries 87

Quinoa Breakfast Bowl with Sautéed Vegetables and a Poached Egg 89

Whole Grain Muffins with Mashed Sweet Potato and Pecans 91

Chia Seed Pudding Topped with Sliced Almonds and Fresh Fruit.. 93

Whole Grain Waffles with Almond Butter and Sliced Strawberries 94

Breakfast Burrito filled with Scrambled Eggs, Black Beans, Avocado, and Salsa 95

LUNCH 96

Quinoa Salad with Chickpeas and Mixed Vegetables 96

Lentil Soup with Spinach and Tomatoes 98

Grilled Chicken and Vegetable Wrap with Whole Grain Tortilla .. 100

Brown Rice Stir-Fry with Tofu and Broccoli 101

Turkey and Black Bean Chili with Whole Grain Cornbread......... 103

Greek Salad with Mixed Greens, Cucumber, Tomato, Feta, and Chickpeas.. 106

Whole Wheat Pasta Primavera with Grilled Shrimp 108

DINNER 110

Roasted Vegetable and Barley Pilaf.. 110

Bean and Vegetable Burrito Bowls 111

Spinach and Feta Stuffed Chicken Breast with Quinoa Pilaf........ 113

Lentil Soup with Whole Grain Bread.. 115

Chickpea Curry with Brown Rice 117

Turkey and Black Bean Chili with Cornbread 119

Grilled Chicken Salad with Mixed Greens, Avocado, and Beans . 122

DESSERTS 124

Fruit Salad with Melons, Berries, and a Squeeze of Lime Juice ... 124

Banana Oatmeal Cookies made with Mashed Bananas and Oats . 125

Baked Apples with Cinnamon and a Sprinkle of Oats 126

Greek Yogurt with Honey and Sliced Strawberries....................... 128

Poached Pears with a Drizzle of Dark Chocolate Sauce 129

SOUPS AND STEWS.. 130

Lentil Stew 130

Turkey Chili 132

Minestrone Soup 134

Split Pea Soup 135

Beef and Barley Stew 137

CONCLUSION 139

INTRODUCTION

Diverticulitis is a common condition characterized by the inflammation or infection of small pouches called diverticula that form along the walls of the colon.

These pouches typically develop due to increased pressure within the colon, which can cause weak spots in the wall to bulge outward.

While diverticulosis refers to the presence of these pouches without inflammation or infection, diverticulitis occurs when one or more of them become inflamed or infected, leading to symptoms such as fever, nausea, abdominal pain, and changes in bowel habits.

Diet exercises a vital role in controlling diverticulitis and preventing flare-ups.

The primary focus of the diverticulitis diet is to reduce the risk of irritation and inflammation in the colon, thereby alleviating symptoms and promoting healing.

One of the key dietary recommendations is to increase fiber intake. High-fiber foods help soften stool and promote regular bowel movements, reducing the risk of constipation and straining, which can exacerbate diverticulitis symptoms.

In addition to fiber, adequate fluid intake is essential for maintaining bowel regularity and preventing constipation.

Drinking plenty of water throughout the day can help soften stool and make it easier to pass, reducing pressure on the colon walls and lowering the risk of diverticulitis flare-ups.

While fiber-rich foods are generally recommended, you experiencing acute diverticulitis flare-ups may initially benefit from a low-fiber or clear liquid diet to give the colon time to rest and heal.

As symptoms improve, gradually reintroducing fiber-rich foods can help prevent future episodes.

Furthermore, avoiding certain foods that may aggravate diverticulitis symptoms is important.

These include processed foods high in refined sugars and unhealthy fats, spicy foods, and seeds or nuts that may become lodged in the diverticula and cause irritation.

CHAPTER 1

6 COMMON RISK FACTORS THAT LEAD TO THE DEVELOPMENT OF DIVERTICULITIS

1. **Low-fiber diet:** A diet low in fiber is one of the primary risk factors for diverticulitis. Insufficient fiber intake leads to constipation and hard stools, increasing pressure within the colon. This elevated pressure can contribute to the formation of diverticula, small pouches that protrude through weak spots in the colon wall, ultimately leading to diverticulitis when these pouches become inflamed or infected.

2. **Age:** Advancing age is associated with an increased risk of developing diverticulitis. As individuals age, the walls of the colon may weaken, making them more susceptible to the formation of diverticula. Additionally, age-related changes in bowel function, such as decreased motility and reduced elasticity of the colon, can contribute to the development of diverticulitis.

3. **Obesity:** Excess body weight, particularly abdominal fat, can increase intra-abdominal pressure, contributing to the development of diverticula and increasing the risk of inflammation and infection. Furthermore, obesity is often associated with a diet high in processed foods and low in fiber, further exacerbating the risk of diverticulitis.

4. **Lack of physical activity:** Sedentary lifestyle habits, such as lack of regular exercise and prolonged sitting, are associated with an increased risk of diverticulitis. Physical activity helps promote bowel regularity and prevent constipation by stimulating intestinal motility. In contrast, a lack of physical activity can lead to sluggish bowel movements, increasing the likelihood of diverticula formation and subsequent inflammation.

5. **Smoking:** Smoking is a modifiable risk factor that has been linked to an increased risk of diverticulitis. Cigarette smoking has been shown to impair blood flow to the colon, weaken the colon wall, and disrupt the balance of gut bacteria, all of which can

contribute to the development and progression of diverticular disease.

6. **Genetics:** Family history and genetic factors also play a role in the development of diverticulitis. Individuals with a family history of diverticular disease are at higher risk of developing the condition themselves. While the exact genetic mechanisms underlying diverticulitis are not fully understood, genetic predisposition likely interacts with environmental factors to influence disease susceptibility.

SIMPLE STRATEGIES FOR RELIEVING SYMPTOMS

1. **Increase fiber intake:** Gradually add high-fiber foods such as fruits, vegetables, whole grains, and legumes to your diet to promote regular bowel movements and prevent constipation.
2. **Stay hydrated:** Drink plenty of water throughout the day to soften stool and ease bowel movements, reducing pressure on the colon walls.

3. **Avoid trigger foods:** Identify and avoid foods that worsen symptoms, such as spicy foods, processed foods, and seeds or nuts that may irritate diverticula.
4. **Limit red meat and fatty foods:** Reduce consumption of red meat and high-fat foods, which can be harder to digest and may exacerbate symptoms.
5. **Eat smaller, more frequent meals:** Go for smaller, more frequent meals to ease digestion and prevent overloading the colon.
6. **Try a low-residue diet during flare-ups:** During acute flare-ups, follow a low-residue or clear liquid diet to rest the colon and alleviate symptoms.
7. **Use over-the-counter pain relievers:** Over-the-counter pain relievers such as acetaminophen or ibuprofen can help alleviate abdominal pain associated with diverticulitis. However, it is advisable to consult a healthcare personnel for proper medication prescription.
8. **Apply heat:** Applying a heating pad or warm compress to the abdomen can help relieve discomfort and relax abdominal muscles.

9. **Practice stress-reduction techniques:** Engage in stress-reduction techniques such as deep breathing, meditation, yoga, or tai chi to help manage stress, which can exacerbate symptoms.
10. **Get regular exercise:** Engage in regular physical activity to promote bowel regularity, reduce constipation, and improve overall gastrointestinal health.
11. **Consider probiotics:** Probiotic supplements or probiotic-rich foods such as yogurt may help restore a healthy balance of gut bacteria and alleviate symptoms.
12. **Avoid smoking:** If you smoke, quitting smoking can help improve blood flow to the colon, reduce inflammation, and decrease the risk of diverticulitis complications.
13. **Practice good bathroom habits:** Avoid delaying or straining during bowel movements, as this can increase pressure on the colon and worsen symptoms.

14. **Stay informed:** Educate yourself about diverticulitis, its triggers, and management strategies to better understand and cope with the condition.
15. **Follow up with healthcare provider:** Regularly follow up with your healthcare provider to monitor your condition, discuss treatment options, and make any necessary adjustments to your management plan.

FOODS TO AVOID FOR DIVERTICULITIS PATIENTS

1. **Seeds and nuts:** Foods like popcorn, sunflower seeds, and peanuts can get lodged in diverticula, leading to irritation and inflammation of the colon.
2. **Processed meats:** Deli meats, bacon, sausage, and other processed meats are high in fat and additives, which can exacerbate diverticulitis symptoms and increase inflammation.
3. **Spicy foods:** Spicy foods can irritate the digestive tract and trigger flare-ups of diverticulitis symptoms such as abdominal pain and discomfort.

4. **Fried foods:** Fried foods are high in unhealthy fats, which can be difficult to digest and may worsen symptoms of diverticulitis.
5. **High-fat dairy:** Full-fat dairy products like whole milk, cheese, and ice cream can be hard to digest and may contribute to inflammation in the colon.
6. **Red meat:** Red meat, especially fatty cuts like steak and ground beef, can be difficult to digest and may increase the risk of diverticulitis flare-ups.
7. **Refined grains:** Processed grains like white bread, white rice, and pasta lack fiber and nutrients, which are essential for maintaining digestive health and preventing diverticulitis.
8. **Sugary foods and beverages:** Foods and drinks high in added sugars can disrupt gut bacteria balance and contribute to inflammation, worsening diverticulitis symptoms.
9. **Alcohol:** Alcohol can cause an irritation to the digestive tract that can lead to dehydration, which can lead symptoms of diverticulitis.

10. **Carbonated beverages:** Carbonated beverages can cause gas and bloating, which may increase discomfort in individuals with diverticulitis.
11. **Caffeine:** Caffeinated beverages like coffee, tea, and energy drinks can stimulate the digestive tract and may worsen symptoms of diverticulitis in some individuals.
12. **Raw vegetables:** Raw vegetables with tough skins or seeds, such as cucumbers, tomatoes, and bell peppers, can be difficult to digest and may cause irritation in the colon.
13. **Dried fruits:** Dried fruits like raisins, apricots, and prunes are concentrated sources of fiber and may be too rough on the digestive system for some individuals with diverticulitis.
14. **Spelt and bran:** While high in fiber, spelt and bran can be too abrasive for inflamed intestines and may exacerbate diverticulitis symptoms.
15. **Corn and mushrooms:** Corn kernels and mushrooms can be hard to digest and may cause irritation in individuals with diverticulitis. It is advisable to avoid them, mostly during flare-ups.

THE 3 SYMPTOM-SPECIFIC STEPS DIET

The 3 Symptom-Specific Steps Diet is a dietary approach designed to manage diverticulitis by gradually transitioning through different phases based on symptom severity and stage of the condition. Each step focuses on specific dietary modifications aimed at alleviating symptoms, promoting healing, and preventing complications. These steps include the Clear Liquid Diet, Low Fiber Diet, and High Fiber Diet.

STEP 1: CLEAR LIQUID DIET

The Clear Liquid Diet is the initial phase of the Symptom-Specific Steps Diet and is typically recommended during acute diverticulitis flare-ups or when symptoms are severe. This phase focuses on consuming easily digestible liquids that leave minimal residue in the digestive tract, giving the colon time to rest and heal. Clear liquids include:

- **Water:** To stay hydrated, drink a good quantity of plain water throughout the day. Adequate hydration helps soften stool and prevent constipation.

- **Broth:** Clear, fat-free broths such as chicken or vegetable broth provide essential fluids and electrolytes to prevent dehydration.
- **Fruit juices:** Go for clear fruit juices without pulp, such as apple juice or white grape juice. These provide energy and hydration without adding fiber.
- **Gelatin:** Clear gelatin desserts or fruit-flavored gelatin cups can provide a source of calories and hydration during the Clear Liquid Diet phase.
- **Clear sports drinks:** Electrolyte-rich sports drinks helps in replenishing electrolytes lost due to vomiting or diarrhea.

During the Clear Liquid Diet phase, it's essential to avoid solid foods, dairy products, and beverages with pulp or residue, as they can be harder to digest and may exacerbate symptoms. The goal of this phase is to rest the digestive system, alleviate inflammation, and prepare for the gradual reintroduction of solid foods.

STEP 2: LOW FIBER DIET

After symptoms have improved and the acute phase of diverticulitis has passed, the Low Fiber Diet phase focuses on reintroducing solid foods while still limiting fiber intake to prevent irritation of the colon. This phase typically includes:

- **Cooked vegetables:** Steamed or boiled vegetables without skins or seeds, such as carrots, squash, and green beans, are easier to digest than raw vegetables.
- **Ripe fruits:** Soft, ripe fruits without seeds or skins, such as bananas, applesauce, and melons, are gentle on the digestive system.
- **White bread and refined grains:** Choose white bread, white rice, and refined pasta over whole grains, which are lower in fiber and easier to digest.
- **Lean proteins:** Go for lean sources of protein such as poultry, fish, eggs, and tofu, which are less likely to cause irritation in the colon.
- **Low-fiber snacks:** Choose low-fiber snacks such as plain crackers, pretzels, or rice cakes to satisfy hunger between meals.

STEP 3: HIGH FIBER DIET

Once symptoms have subsided and the colon has had time to heal, the High Fiber Diet phase focuses on gradually increasing fiber intake to promote regular bowel movements, prevent constipation, and reduce the risk of diverticulitis recurrence. This phase includes:

- **Whole grains:** Incorporate whole grains such as whole wheat bread, brown rice, quinoa, and oats into your diet to increase fiber intake.
- **Fruits and vegetables:** Include a variety of fruits and vegetables with skins and seeds, such as berries, broccoli, spinach, and sweet potatoes, to provide a rich source of dietary fiber.
- **Legumes:** Add legumes such as beans, lentils, and chickpeas to soups, salads, and stews to boost fiber content and promote digestive health.
- **Nuts and seeds:** Enjoy small portions of nuts and seeds as snacks or toppings for salads and yogurt to add healthy fats and fiber to your diet.
- **Hydration:** Drink plenty of water throughout the day to help soften stool and prevent constipation, especially when increasing fiber intake.

CHAPTER 2

NUTRITIOUS RECIPES FOR A DIVERTICULITIS DIET

CLEAR LIQUID DIET FOR FLARE UPS

BREAKFAST

Vegetable Broth

Preparation time: 1 hour

Serves: 2

Calories: 45 **Carbs:** 10g **Protein:** 1g **Fat:** 0g **Fiber:** 2g **Sodium:** 100mg

Ingredients:

4 cups water

1 onion, chopped

2 carrots, chopped

2 celery stalks, chopped

1 parsnip, chopped

1 small potato, chopped

1 bay leaf

A pinch of salt

Method of Preparation:

1. In a large pot, bring water to a boil over medium heat.
2. Add chopped onion, carrots, celery, parsnip, potato, and bay leaf to the pot.
3. Reduce heat to low and simmer for 45 minutes to 1 hour, until vegetables are tender.
4. Remove the pot from heat and let cool slightly.
5. Strain the broth through a fine mesh sieve or cheesecloth into a clean container.
6. Discard the solids and season the broth with A pinch of salt.
7. Serve hot.

Clear Herbal Tea

Preparation time: 10 minutes

Serves: 2

Calories: 0 **Carbs:** 0g **Protein:** 0g **Fat:** 0g **Fiber:** 0g **Sodium:** 0mg

Ingredients:

2 cups water

2 herbal tea bags (chamomile, peppermint, or ginger)

Method of Preparation:

1. Bring water to a boil in a small saucepan.
2. Remove the saucepan from heat and add herbal tea bags.
3. Cover the saucepan and let steep for 5-7 minutes.
4. Remove the tea bags and discard.
5. Pour the herbal tea into cups and serve hot.

Coconut Water

Preparation time: 2 minutes

Serves: 2

Calories: 45 **Carbs:** 10g **Protein:** 1g **Fat:** 0g **Fiber:** 0g **Sodium:** 60mg

Ingredients:

2 cups coconut water

Method of Preparation:

1. Chill coconut water in the refrigerator or serve over ice cubes.
2. Pour coconut water into glasses and serve immediately.

Clear Sports Drink

Preparation time: 5 minutes

Serves: 2

Calories: 70 **Carbs:** 19g **Protein:** 0g **Fat:** 0g **Fiber:** 0g **Sodium:** 90mg

Ingredients:

2 cups water

1/4 teaspoon salt

2 tablespoons honey or maple syrup

1/4 cup fresh lemon juice

Method of Preparation:

1. In a pitcher, combine water, salt, honey or maple syrup, and fresh lemon juice.
2. Stir until the salt and sweetener are dissolved.
3. Chill in the refrigerator before serving or pour over ice cubes.
4. Serve cold.

Blueberry, Spinach and Banana Smoothie

Preparation time: 5 minutes

Serves: 2

Calories: 90 **Carbs:** 22g **Protein:** 2g **Fat:** 0g **Fiber:** 4g **Sodium:** 90mg

Ingredients:

1 cup fresh spinach leaves

1 ripe banana, peeled

1/2 cup fresh or frozen blueberries

1 cup coconut water (unsweetened)

Method of Preparation:

1. Place spinach leaves, banana, blueberries, and coconut water in a blender.
2. Blend until smooth and creamy.
3. If desired, add ice cubes for a colder smoothie.
4. Pour into glasses and serve immediately.

Apple Flavored Popsicles

Preparation time: 5 minutes + freezing time

Serves: 2

Calories: 70 **Carbs:** 18g **Protein:** 0g **Fat:** 0g **Fiber:** 0g **Sodium:** 10mg

Ingredients:

2 cups unsweetened apple juice

1/2 cup water

1 tablespoon honey or maple syrup (optional)

Method of Preparation:

1. In a bowl, mix unsweetened apple juice, water, and honey or maple syrup (if using) until well combined.

2. Pour the mixture into popsicle molds.
3. Insert popsicle sticks into each mold.
4. Place the molds in the freezer and freeze for at least 4 hours or until solid.
5. Once frozen, remove the popsicles from the molds and serve immediately.

Clear Protein Drink

Preparation time: 2 minutes

Serves: 2

Calories: 60 **Carbs:** 1g **Protein:** 15g **Fat:** 0g **Fiber:** 0g **Sodium:** 45mg

Ingredients:

1 cup water

1 scoop unflavored protein powder (whey or plant-based)

1/2 teaspoon honey or maple syrup (optional)

Method of Preparation:

1. In a shaker bottle or blender, combine water and unflavored protein powder.

2. Add honey or maple syrup (if using) for sweetness.
3. Shake or blend until well combined and frothy.
4. Pour into glasses and serve immediately.

LUNCH

Chicken Broth

Preparation time: 1.5 hours

Serves: 2

Calories: 100 **Carbs:** 5g **Protein:** 15g **Fat:** 2g **Fiber:** 1g **Sodium:** 100mg

Ingredients:

4 cups water

1 boneless, skinless chicken breast (about 8 ounces)

1 onion, quartered

2 carrots, chopped

2 celery stalks, chopped

1 bay leaf

A pinch of salt

Method of Preparation:

1. In a large pot, combine water, chicken breast, onion, carrots, celery, and bay leaf.
2. Bring to a boil over medium-high heat.
3. Reduce heat to low, cover, and simmer for 1 to 1.5 hours, until the chicken is cooked through and tender.
4. Remove the chicken breast from the pot and set aside to cool slightly.
5. Strain the broth through a fine mesh sieve or cheesecloth into a clean container.
6. Discard the solids and season the broth with a pinch of salt.
7. Shred or chop the cooked chicken breast and add it back to the broth, if desired.
8. Serve hot.

Clear Vegetable Soup

Preparation time: 45 minutes

Serves: 2

Calories: 60 **Carbs:** 15g **Protein:** 3g **Fat:** 0g **Fiber:** 5g **Sodium:** 100mg

Ingredients:

4 cups water

1 onion, chopped

2 carrots, chopped

2 celery stalks, chopped

1 zucchini, chopped

1 cup spinach leaves

1 bay leaf

A pinch of salt

Method of Preparation:

1. In a large pot, bring water to a boil over medium heat.
2. Add chopped onion, carrots, celery, zucchini, spinach, and bay leaf to the pot.
3. Reduce heat to low and simmer for 30-45 minutes, until vegetables are tender.
4. Remove the bay leaf from the pot and discard.
5. Season the soup with a pinch of salt.
6. Serve hot.

Clear Fish Broth

Preparation time: 1 hour

Serves: 2

Calories: 50 **Carbs:** 5g **Protein:** 10g **Fat:** 1g **Fiber:** 1g **Sodium:** 100mg

Ingredients:

4 cups water

1 pound fish bones or fish heads (cleaned and rinsed)

1 onion, chopped

2 carrots, chopped

2 celery stalks, chopped

1 bay leaf

A pinch of salt

Method of Preparation:

1. In a large pot, combine water, fish bones or heads, onion, carrots, celery, and bay leaf.
2. Bring to a boil over medium-high heat.

3. Reduce heat to low, cover, and simmer for 1 hour.
4. Remove the pot from heat and let cool slightly.
5. Strain the broth through a fine mesh sieve or cheesecloth into a clean container.
6. Discard the solids and season the broth with a pinch of salt.
7. Serve hot.

Apple Juice

Preparation time: 10 minutes

Serves: 2

Calories: 60 **Carbs:** 15g **Protein:** 0g **Fat:** 0g **Fiber:** 2g **Sodium:** 0mg

Ingredients:

2 apples

2 cups water

Method of Preparation:

1. Wash and core the apples, then chop them into small pieces.
2. In a blender, combine chopped apples and water.

3. Blend until smooth.
4. Strain the mixture through a fine mesh sieve or cheesecloth into a clean container to remove pulp.
5. Discard the pulp.
6. Chill the apple juice in the refrigerator before serving or pour over ice cubes.
7. Serve cold.

Beef Soup

Preparation time: 2 hours

Serves: 2

Calories: 200 **Carbs:** 10g **Protein:** 25g **Fat:** 7g **Fiber:** 2g **Sodium:** 100mg

Ingredients:

4 cups water

8 ounces lean beef (such as sirloin or round), cut into cubes

1 onion, chopped

2 carrots, chopped

2 celery stalks, chopped

1 bay leaf

A pinch of salt

Method of Preparation:

1. In a large pot, bring water to a boil over medium-high heat.
2. Add lean beef cubes, chopped onion, carrots, celery, and bay leaf to the pot.
3. Reduce heat to low, cover, and simmer for 1.5 to 2 hours, until the beef is tender.
4. Remove the pot from heat and let cool slightly.
5. Skim off any excess fat from the surface of the soup, if necessary.
6. Season the soup with a pinch of salt.
7. Serve hot.

Gelatin Desserts

Preparation time: 10 minutes + chilling time

Serves: 2

Calories: 20 **Carbs:** 1g **Protein:** 5g **Fat:** 0g **Fiber:** 0g **Sodium:** 20mg

Ingredients:

1 packet unflavored gelatin

1 cup water

1 tablespoon honey or maple syrup (optional)

Method of Preparation:

1. In a small saucepan, sprinkle unflavored gelatin over water and let it soften for 5 minutes.
2. Place the saucepan over low heat and stir until the gelatin is completely dissolved.
3. Remove from heat and stir in honey or maple syrup (if using) until well combined.
4. Pour the mixture into individual serving cups or molds.
5. Chill in the refrigerator for at least 2 hours, until set.
6. Serve chilled.

Apple, Pear, and Carrot Smoothie

Preparation time: 5 minutes

Serves: 2

Calories: 80 **Carbs:** 20g **Protein:** 1g **Fat:** 0g **Fiber:** 5gm **Sodium:** 100mg

Ingredients:

1 apple, cored and chopped

1 pear, cored and chopped

1 carrot, peeled and chopped

1 cup coconut water (unsweetened)

Method of Preparation:

1. Place chopped apple, pear, carrot, and coconut water in a blender.
2. Blend until smooth and creamy.
3. If desired, add ice cubes for a colder smoothie.
4. Pour into glasses and serve immediately.

DINNER

Clear Beef Broth

Preparation time: 2 hours

Serves: 2

Calories: 100 **Carbs:** 5g **Protein:** 15g **Fat:** 2g **Fiber:** 1g **Sodium:** 100mg

Ingredients:

4 cups water

8 ounces lean beef (such as sirloin or round), cut into cubes

1 onion, chopped

2 carrots, chopped

2 celery stalks, chopped

1 bay leaf

A pinch of salt

Method of Preparation:

1. In a large pot, bring water to a boil over medium-high heat.
2. Add lean beef cubes, chopped onion, carrots, celery, and bay leaf to the pot.
3. Reduce heat to low, cover, and simmer for 1.5 to 2 hours, until the beef is tender.
4. Remove the pot from heat and let cool slightly.

5. Skim off any excess fat from the surface of the broth, if necessary.
6. Season the broth with a pinch of salt.
7. Strain the broth through a fine mesh sieve or cheesecloth into a clean container.
8. Discard the solids and serve hot.

Clear Miso Soup

Preparation time: 15 minutes

Serves: 2

Calories: 60 **Carbs:** 8g **Protein:** 5g **Fat:** 2g **Fiber:** 2g **Sodium:** 100mg

Ingredients:

4 cups water

3 tablespoons white miso paste

2 green onions, thinly sliced

1/2 cup tofu, diced

1/2 cup seaweed (such as wakame), rehydrated and chopped (optional)

Method of Preparation:

1. In a medium saucepan, bring water to a simmer over medium heat.
2. Place miso paste in a small bowl and gradually whisk in a small amount of hot water until smooth.
3. Add the diluted miso paste to the simmering water in the saucepan.
4. Stir in sliced green onions, diced tofu, and rehydrated seaweed (if using).
5. Simmer for 5-7 minutes, until heated through.
6. Remove from heat and let cool slightly.
7. Serve hot.

Clear Chicken Noodle Soup (Strained)

Preparation time: 1.5 hours

Serves: 2

Calories: 100 **Carbs:** 5g **Protein:** 15g **Fat:** 2g **Fiber:** 1g **Sodium:** 100mg

Ingredients:

4 cups water

1 boneless, skinless chicken breast (about 8 ounces)

1 onion, chopped

2 carrots, chopped

2 celery stalks, chopped

1 bay leaf

A pinch of salt

Cooked egg noodles (optional)

Method of Preparation:

1. In a large pot, combine water, chicken breast, chopped onion, carrots, celery, and bay leaf.
2. Bring to a boil over medium-high heat.
3. Reduce heat to low, cover, and simmer for 1 to 1.5 hours, until the chicken is cooked through and tender.
4. Remove the chicken breast from the pot and set aside to cool slightly.
5. Strain the soup through a fine mesh sieve or cheesecloth into a clean container.

6. Discard the solids and season the strained soup with a pinch of salt.
7. Shred or chop the cooked chicken breast and add it back to the strained soup, if desired.
8. Serve hot, with cooked egg noodles if desired.

Fruit Juice Gelatin

Preparation time: 10 minutes + chilling time

Serves: 2

Calories: 40 **Carbs:** 10g **Protein:** 1g **Fat:** 0g **Fiber:** 0g **Sodium:** 0mg

Ingredients:

1 packet unflavored gelatin

1 cup fruit juice (such as apple or pear juice)

1 tablespoon honey or maple syrup (optional)

Method of Preparation:

1. In a small saucepan, sprinkle unflavored gelatin over fruit juice and let it soften for 5 minutes.

2. Place the saucepan over low heat and stir until the gelatin is completely dissolved.
3. Remove from heat and stir in honey or maple syrup (if using) until well combined.
4. Pour the mixture into individual serving cups or molds.
5. Chill in the refrigerator for at least 2 hours, until set.
6. Serve chilled.

Clear Chicken Soup

Preparation time: 1.5 hours

Serves: 2

Calories: 100 **Carbs:** 5g **Protein:** 15g **Fat:** 2g **Fiber:** 1g **Sodium:** 100mg

Ingredients:

4 cups water

1 boneless, skinless chicken breast (about 8 ounces)

1 onion, chopped

2 carrots, chopped

2 celery stalks, chopped

1 bay leaf

A pinch of salt

Method of Preparation:

1. In a large pot, combine water, chicken breast, chopped onion, carrots, celery, and bay leaf.
2. Bring to a boil over medium-high heat.
3. Reduce heat to low, cover, and simmer for 1 to 1.5 hours, until the chicken is cooked through and tender.
4. Remove the chicken breast from the pot and set aside to cool slightly.
5. Strain the soup through a fine mesh sieve or cheesecloth into a clean container.
6. Discard the solids and season the strained soup with A pinch of salt.
7. Shred or chop the cooked chicken breast and add it back to the strained soup, if desired.
8. Serve hot.

White Grape Juice

Preparation time: 2 minutes

Serves: 2

Calories: 120 **Carbs:** 30g **Protein:** 1g **Fat:** 0g **Fiber:** 0g **Sodium:** 10mg

Ingredients:

2 cups white grape juice

Method of Preparation:

1. Chill white grape juice in the refrigerator or serve over ice cubes.
2. Pour white grape juice into glasses and serve immediately.

Clear Strained Fruit Juice

Preparation time: 10 minutes

Serves: 2

Calories: 100 **Carbs:** 25g **Protein:** 1g **Fat:** 0g **Fiber:** 1g **Sodium:** 10mg

Ingredients:

2 cups mixed fruit (such as apple, pear, and pineapple)

2 cups water

Cheesecloth or fine mesh sieve

Method of Preparation:

1. Wash and chop the mixed fruit into small pieces, removing any seeds or pits.
2. Place chopped fruit and water in a blender and blend until smooth.
3. Strain the fruit mixture through a cheesecloth or fine mesh sieve into a clean container to remove pulp.
4. Discard the pulp and pour the strained fruit juice into glasses.
5. Chill in the refrigerator before serving or pour over ice cubes.
6. Serve cold.

LOW FIBER DIET

BREAKFAST

Refined Oatmeal with Sliced Strawberries

Preparation time: 10 minutes

Serves: 2

Calories: 150 **Carbs:** 30g **Protein:** 3g **Fat:** 1g **Fiber:** 4g **Sodium:** 0mg

Ingredients:

1/2 cup refined oatmeal

1 cup water

1/2 cup sliced strawberries

Method of Preparation:

1. In a small saucepan, bring water to a boil over medium heat.
2. Add refined oatmeal to the boiling water and stir.

3. Reduce heat to low and simmer for 5-7 minutes, stirring occasionally, until oatmeal is cooked and reaches desired consistency.
4. Remove from heat and let cool slightly.
5. Serve the cooked oatmeal topped with sliced strawberries.

Cucumber Smoothie with Plain Yogurt

Preparation time: 5 minutes

Serves: 2

Calories: 80 **Carbs:** 10g **Protein:** 6g **Fat:** 2g **Fiber:** 1g **Sodium:** 50mg

Ingredients:

1 cucumber, peeled and chopped

1 cup plain yogurt (unsweetened)

1/2 cup water

Honey or maple syrup, to taste (optional)

Ice cubes (optional)

Method of Preparation:

1. In a blender, combine chopped cucumber, plain yogurt, and water.
2. Add honey or maple syrup (if using) for sweetness.
3. Blend until smooth and creamy.
4. If desired, add ice cubes for a colder smoothie.
5. Pour into glasses and serve immediately.

Egg White Omelet with Cooked Carrots

Preparation time: 10 minutes

Serves: 2

Calories: 70 **Carbs:** 5g **Protein:** 13g **Fat:** 0g **Fiber:** 1g **Sodium:** 150mg

Ingredients:

4 egg whites

1/2 cup cooked carrots, chopped

A pinch of salt and pepper

Cooking spray or olive oil (for greasing pan)

Method of Preparation:

1. In a bowl, whisk together egg whites until frothy.
2. Heat a non-stick skillet over medium heat and lightly coat with cooking spray or olive oil.
3. Pour the whisked egg whites into the skillet.
4. Sprinkle chopped cooked carrots evenly over the egg whites.
5. Cook until the edges start to set, then gently lift the edges with a spatula and tilt the skillet to allow the uncooked egg to flow underneath.
6. Once the omelet is set, fold it in half and cook for another minute.
7. Season with A pinch of salt and pepper.
8. Serve hot.

Plain Yogurt with Mashed Ripe Banana

Preparation time: 5 minutes

Serves: 2

Calories: 150 **Carbs:** 25g **Protein:** 7g **Fat:** 3g **Fiber:** 2g **Sodium:** 100mg

Ingredients:

1 cup plain yogurt (unsweetened)

1 ripe banana, mashed

Method of Preparation:

1. In a bowl, combine plain yogurt and mashed ripe banana.
2. Mix until well combined.
3. Serve immediately.

Scrambled Eggs with Well-Cooked Spinach

Preparation time: 10 minutes

Serves: 2

Calories: 160 **Carbs:** 2g **Protein:** 14g **Fat:** 10g **Fiber:** 1g **Sodium:** 220mg

Ingredients:

4 large eggs

1 cup well-cooked spinach, chopped

A pinch of salt and pepper

Method of Preparation:

1. In a bowl, whisk together eggs until well beaten.
2. In a non-stick skillet, add the beaten eggs and cook over medium heat.
3. As the eggs begin to set, gently fold in the chopped well-cooked spinach.
4. Continue cooking until the eggs are fully cooked and the spinach is heated through.
5. Season with A pinch of salt and pepper.
6. Serve hot.

White Toast with Creamy Peanut Butter

Preparation time: 5 minutes

Serves: 2

Calories: 260 **Carbs:** 22g **Protein:** 10g **Fat:** 15g **Fiber:** 2g **Sodium:** 50mg

Ingredients:

2 slices white bread (toasted)

2 tablespoons creamy peanut butter

Method of Preparation:

1. Toast the white bread slices until golden brown.
2. Spread 1 tablespoon of creamy peanut butter onto each slice of toast.
3. Serve immediately.

Poached Eggs on White Toast with Peeled and Cooked Tomatoes

Preparation time: 15 minutes

Serves: 2

Calories: 200 **Carbs:** 20g **Protein:** 12g **Fat:** 7g **Fiber:** 3g **Sodium:** 150mg

Ingredients:

2 eggs

2 slices white bread (toasted)

2 tomatoes, peeled and cooked

A pinch of salt and pepper

Vinegar (optional, for poaching)

Method of Preparation:

1. Fill a medium saucepan with water and bring it to a gentle simmer over medium heat.
2. Crack one egg into a small bowl or ramekin.
3. If desired, add a splash of vinegar to the simmering water (this helps the egg whites to set).
4. Carefully slide the egg into the simmering water and let it cook for 3-4 minutes, until the whites are set but the yolk is still runny.
5. Use a slotted spoon to carefully remove the poached egg from the water and drain excess water.
6. Repeat the process with the second egg.
7. Place a slice of toasted white bread on each plate.
8. Top each slice of toast with a peeled and cooked tomato.
9. Carefully place a poached egg on top of each tomato.
10. Season with A pinch of salt and pepper.
11. Serve immediately.

Rice Cakes with Cream Cheese and Sliced Avocado

Preparation time: 5 minutes

Serves: 2

Calories: 200 **Carbs:** 18g **Protein:** 3g **Fat:** 14g **Fiber:** 5g **Sodium:** 80mg

Ingredients:

2 rice cakes

2 tablespoons cream cheese

1 avocado, sliced

A pinch of salt and pepper

Method of Preparation:

1. Spread 1 tablespoon of cream cheese onto each rice cake.
2. Top each rice cake with sliced avocado.
3. Season with A pinch of salt and pepper.
4. Serve immediately.

LUNCH

Chicken and Rice Soup

Preparation time: 30 minutes

Serves: 2

Calories: 250 **Carbs:** 25g **Protein:** 20g **Fat:** 7g **Fiber:** 2g **Sodium:** 60mg

Ingredients:

4 cups chicken broth (low sodium)

1 boneless, skinless chicken breast (about 8 ounces), cooked and shredded

1/2 cup white rice

1 carrot, diced

1 celery stalk, diced

A pinch of salt and pepper

Fresh parsley, chopped (optional, for garnish)

Method of Preparation:

1. In a large pot, bring chicken broth to a boil over medium-high heat.
2. Add shredded chicken breast, white rice, diced carrot, and diced celery to the pot.
3. Reduce heat to low, cover, and simmer for 20-25 minutes, until the rice is cooked and vegetables are tender.
4. Season with A pinch of salt and pepper.
5. Ladle the soup into bowls, garnish with chopped fresh parsley if desired, and serve hot.

Mashed Potatoes with Grilled Chicken Breast

Preparation time: 30 minutes

Serves: 2

Calories: 300 **Carbs:** 30g **Protein:** 25g **Fat:** 8g **Fiber:** 3g **Sodium:** 100mg

Ingredients:

2 small potatoes, peeled and cubed

2 tablespoons milk (or dairy-free alternative)

A pinch of salt and pepper

1 boneless, skinless chicken breast (about 8 ounces), grilled and sliced

Fresh parsley, chopped (optional, for garnish)

Method of Preparation:

1. Place potato cubes in a pot of boiling water and cook until tender, about 15 minutes.
2. Drain the potatoes and transfer them to a mixing bowl.
3. Add milk, salt, and pepper to the potatoes and mash until smooth and creamy.
4. Serve the mashed potatoes topped with grilled chicken breast slices.
5. Garnish with chopped fresh parsley if desired and serve hot.

Tuna Salad on White Bread

Preparation time: 10 minutes

Serves: 2

Calories: 300 **Carbs:** 25g **Protein:** 20g **Fat:** 15g **Fiber:** 2g **Sodium:** 50mg

Ingredients:

1 can (5 ounces) tuna, drained

2 tablespoons mayonnaise (or Greek yogurt for a lighter option)

1 tablespoon lemon juice

1 celery stalk, finely chopped

A pinch of salt and pepper

4 slices white bread

Method of Preparation:

1. In a mixing bowl, combine drained tuna, mayonnaise, lemon juice, and chopped celery.
2. Mix until well combined.
3. Season with A pinch of salt and pepper.
4. Divide the tuna salad mixture evenly among the slices of white bread.
5. Serve immediately.

Scrambled Eggs with Soft-Cooked Vegetables

Preparation time: 10 minutes

Serves: 2

Calories: 200 **Carbs:** 5g **Protein:** 14g **Fat:** 14g **Fiber:** 2g **Sodium:** 100mg

Ingredients:

4 eggs

1/2 cup mixed soft-cooked vegetables (such as spinach, bell peppers, and mushrooms), chopped

A pinch of salt and pepper

Cooking spray or olive oil (for greasing pan)

Method of Preparation:

1. In a bowl, whisk together the eggs until well beaten.
2. Heat a non-stick skillet over medium heat and lightly coat with cooking spray or olive oil.
3. Add the mixed soft-cooked vegetables to the skillet and sauté for 2-3 minutes until heated through.

4. Pour the beaten eggs into the skillet over the vegetables.
5. Cook, stirring occasionally, until the eggs are scrambled and fully cooked.
6. Season with A pinch of salt and pepper.
7. Serve hot.

Baked Salmon with Steamed Carrots and White Rice

Preparation time: 20 minutes

Serves: 2

Calories: 350 **Carbs:** 30g **Protein:** 30g **Fat:** 12g **Fiber:** 3g **Sodium:** 100mg

Ingredients:

2 salmon fillets (about 6 ounces each)

A pinch of salt and pepper

1 cup carrots, sliced

1 cup white rice, cooked

Method of Preparation:

1. Preheat the oven to 400°F (200°C).
2. Season the salmon fillets with salt and pepper on both sides.
3. Place the seasoned salmon fillets on a baking sheet lined with parchment paper.
4. Bake in the preheated oven for 12-15 minutes, or until the salmon is cooked through and flakes easily with a fork.
5. While the salmon is baking, steam the sliced carrots until tender, about 5-7 minutes.
6. Serve the baked salmon with steamed carrots and cooked white rice on the side.
7. Serve hot.

Turkey and Cheese Sandwich on White Bread

Preparation time: 5 minutes

Serves: 2

Calories: 300 **Carbs:** 25g **Protein:** 20g **Fat:** 15g **Fiber:** 2g **Sodium:** 100mg

Ingredients:

4 slices white bread

4 slices turkey breast

2 slices cheese

Lettuce leaves

Tomato slices

Mustard or mayonnaise (optional)

Method of Preparation:

1. Place two slices of white bread on a clean surface.
2. Layer each slice of bread with turkey breast, cheese, lettuce leaves, and tomato slices.
3. If desired, spread mustard or mayonnaise on the other two slices of white bread.
4. Place the mustard or mayonnaise spread slices on top of the prepared sandwich fillings.
5. Cut each sandwich in half and serve immediately.

Vegetable Broth with Soft-Cooked Noodles

Preparation time: 15 minutes

Serves: 2

Calories: 150 **Carbs:** 25g **Protein:** 5g **Fat:** 3g **Fiber:** 3g **Sodium:** 60mg

Ingredients:

4 cups vegetable broth (low sodium)

1 cup soft-cooked noodles (such as egg noodles or rice noodles)

1 carrot, sliced

1 celery stalk, sliced

A pinch of salt and pepper

Fresh parsley, chopped (optional, for garnish)

Method of Preparation:

1. In a medium saucepan, bring vegetable broth to a simmer over medium heat.

2. Add sliced carrot and celery to the simmering broth.
3. Simmer for 5-7 minutes until the vegetables are tender.
4. Add the soft-cooked noodles to the broth and stir to combine.
5. Season with A pinch of salt and pepper.
6. Ladle the vegetable broth with soft-cooked noodles into bowls.
7. Garnish with chopped fresh parsley if desired and serve hot.

Salmon Vegetable Soup

Preparation time: 20 minutes

Serves: 2

Calories: 200 **Carbs:** 15g **Protein:** 20g **Fat:** 8g **Fiber:** 4g **Sodium:** 70mg

Ingredients:

4 cups vegetable broth (low sodium)

2 salmon fillets (about 6 ounces each), cooked and flaked

1 cup mixed vegetables (such as carrots, celery, and green beans), diced

A pinch of salt and pepper

Fresh dill, chopped (optional, for garnish)

Method of Preparation:

1. In a large pot, bring vegetable broth to a boil over medium-high heat.
2. Add diced mixed vegetables to the boiling broth.
3. Reduce heat to low, cover, and simmer for 10-12 minutes until the vegetables are tender.
4. Add the cooked and flaked salmon to the pot and simmer for an additional 2-3 minutes until heated through.
5. Season with A pinch of salt and pepper.
6. Ladle the salmon vegetable soup into bowls.
7. Garnish with chopped fresh dill if desired and serve hot.

Plain Pasta with Butter or Olive Oil

Preparation time: 10 minutes

Serves: 2

Calories: 200 **Carbs:** 30g **Protein:** 5g **Fat:** 7g **Fiber:** 2g **Sodium:** 0mg

Ingredients:

1 cup cooked pasta (such as spaghetti or penne)

1 tablespoon butter or olive oil

A pinch of salt and pepper

Fresh parsley, chopped (optional, for garnish)

Method of Preparation:

1. Cook pasta according to package instructions until al dente.
2. Drain the cooked pasta and transfer it to a serving bowl.
3. Add butter or olive oil to the cooked pasta and toss to coat evenly.
4. Season with A pinch of salt and pepper.
5. Garnish with chopped fresh parsley if desired and serve immediately.

DINNER

Baked Cod with Quinoa Pilaf and Steamed Green Beans

Preparation time: 30 minutes

Serves: 2

Calories: 400 **Carbs:** 45g **Protein:** 30g **Fat:** 12g **Fiber:** 8g **Sodium:** 100mg

Ingredients:

2 cod fillets (about 6 ounces each)

A pinch of salt and pepper

1 cup quinoa, rinsed

2 cups water or vegetable broth (low sodium)

1 tablespoon olive oil

1/4 cup diced onion

1/4 cup diced bell pepper

1/4 cup diced carrot

1/4 cup diced zucchini

1/4 cup chopped parsley (optional, for garnish)

1 cup green beans, trimmed

Method of Preparation:

1. Preheat the oven to 375°F (190°C).
2. Season the cod fillets with salt and pepper on both sides.
3. Place the cod fillets on a baking sheet lined with parchment paper.
4. Bake in the preheated oven for 15-20 minutes, or until the cod is cooked through and flakes easily with a fork.
5. While the cod is baking, prepare the quinoa pilaf. In a saucepan, bring water or vegetable broth to a boil.
6. Add quinoa, cover, and simmer for 15-20 minutes, or until the quinoa is cooked and liquid is absorbed.
7. In a separate skillet, heat olive oil over medium heat.
8. Add diced onion, bell pepper, carrot, and zucchini.
9. Cook for 5-7 minutes, or until vegetables are tender.
10. Fluff the cooked quinoa with a fork and stir in the cooked vegetables.

11. Steam green beans until tender, about 5-7 minutes.
12. Serve the baked cod with quinoa pilaf and steamed green beans.
13. Garnish with chopped parsley if desired.

Turkey Chili Made with Ground Turkey, Tomatoes, and Kidney Beans

Preparation time: 40 minutes

Serves: 2

Calories: 400 **Carbs:** 30g **Protein:** 35g **Fat:** 15g **Fiber:** 10g **Sodium:** 50mg

Ingredients:

1 tablespoon olive oil

1/2 onion, diced

1 bell pepper, diced

1 pound ground turkey

1 can (14 ounces) diced tomatoes

1 can (14 ounces) kidney beans, drained and rinsed

1 tablespoon chili powder

1 teaspoon ground cumin

A pinch of salt and pepper

Fresh cilantro, chopped (optional, for garnish)

Method of Preparation:

1. In a large pot, heat olive oil over medium heat.
2. Add diced onion and bell pepper.
3. Cook until softened, about 5-7 minutes.
4. Add ground turkey to the pot and cook until browned, breaking it up with a spoon.
5. Stir in diced tomatoes, kidney beans, chili powder, and ground cumin.
6. Season with salt and pepper to taste.
7. Bring the chili to a simmer, then reduce heat to low.
8. Cover and cook for 20-30 minutes, stirring occasionally.
9. Serve hot, garnished with chopped fresh cilantro if desired.

Roast Chicken with Roasted Sweet Potatoes and Steamed Broccoli

Preparation time: 1.5 hours

Serves: 2

Calories: 500 **Carbs:** 30g **Protein:** 40g **Fat:** 20g **Fiber:** 8g **Sodium:** 30mg

Ingredients:

1 whole chicken (about 3-4 pounds)

A pinch of salt and pepper

2 sweet potatoes, peeled and cubed

1 tablespoon olive oil

2 cups broccoli florets

Method of Preparation:

1. Preheat the oven to 375°F (190°C).
2. Season the whole chicken with salt and pepper, both inside and outside the cavity.
3. Place the seasoned chicken on a roasting pan or baking dish.

4. Arrange the cubed sweet potatoes around the chicken on the roasting pan.
5. Drizzle olive oil over the sweet potatoes and season with salt and pepper.
6. Roast the chicken and sweet potatoes in the preheated oven for 1 to 1.5 hours, or until the chicken is cooked through and golden brown, and the sweet potatoes are tender.
7. While the chicken and sweet potatoes are roasting, steam broccoli florets until tender, about 5-7 minutes.
8. Remove the chicken and sweet potatoes from the oven and let them rest for a few minutes before serving.
9. Serve the roast chicken with roasted sweet potatoes and steamed broccoli.

Beef Stew Made with Tender Beef, Potatoes, and Well-Cooked Carrots

Preparation time: 2.5 hours

Serves: 2

Calories: 500 **Carbs:** 30g **Protein:** 35g **Fat:** 25g **Fiber:** 5g **Sodium:** 70mg

Ingredients:

1 pound beef stew meat, cubed

A pinch of salt and pepper

2 tablespoons olive oil

1 onion, chopped

2 cloves garlic, minced

2 potatoes, peeled and cubed

2 carrots, peeled and sliced

4 cups beef broth (low sodium)

1 bay leaf

Fresh parsley, chopped (optional, for garnish)

Method of Preparation:

1. Season the beef stew meat with salt and pepper.
2. In a large pot, heat olive oil over medium heat.

3. Add the seasoned beef stew meat and cook until browned on all sides.
4. Add chopped onion and minced garlic to the pot. Cook until onions are translucent.
5. Stir in cubed potatoes and sliced carrots.
6. Pour beef broth into the pot and add a bay leaf. Bring to a boil, then reduce heat to low and simmer, covered, for 1.5 to 2 hours, or until beef and vegetables are tender.
7. Remove the bay leaf before serving.
8. Garnish with chopped fresh parsley if desired and serve hot.

Egg Drop Soup with Cooked Chicken and Soft Tofu

Preparation time: 15 minutes

Serves: 2

Calories: 200 **Carbs:** 5g **Protein:** 20g **Fat:** 10g **Fiber:** 1g **Sodium:** 60mg

Ingredients:

4 cups chicken broth (low sodium)

1 cup cooked chicken breast, shredded

1/2 cup soft tofu, cubed

2 eggs, beaten

2 green onions, chopped

A pinch of salt and pepper

Method of Preparation:

1. In a pot, bring chicken broth to a simmer over medium heat.
2. Add shredded cooked chicken breast and cubed soft tofu to the simmering broth.
3. Slowly pour beaten eggs into the simmering soup while stirring gently to create egg ribbons.
4. Season with A pinch of salt and pepper.
5. Cook for another 2-3 minutes until eggs are cooked through.
6. Garnish with chopped green onions before serving.
7. Serve hot.

Vegetable Stir-Fry with Tofu and White Rice

Preparation time: 25 minutes

Serves: 2

Calories: 400 **Carbs:** 40g **Protein:** 20g **Fat:** 15g **Fiber:** 8g **Sodium:** 50mg

Ingredients:

1 cup firm tofu, cubed

2 tablespoons soy sauce (low sodium)

1 tablespoon olive oil

2 cups mixed vegetables (such as bell peppers, broccoli, and snap peas), chopped

Cooked white rice, for serving

Sesame seeds (optional, for garnish)

Method of Preparation:

1. Marinate cubed tofu in soy sauce for 10-15 minutes.

2. Heat olive oil in a skillet over medium heat. Add marinated tofu cubes and cook until golden brown on all sides. Remove tofu from the skillet and set aside.
3. In the same skillet, add chopped mixed vegetables. Stir-fry for 5-7 minutes until vegetables are tender-crisp.
4. Return cooked tofu to the skillet and toss with the vegetables.
5. Serve vegetable stir-fry over cooked white rice.
6. Garnish with sesame seeds if desired and serve hot.

Baked Chicken Breast with Mashed Potatoes and Steamed Carrots

Preparation time: 40 minutes

Serves: 2

Calories: 400 **Carbs:** 30g **Protein:** 40g **Fat:** 10g **Fiber:** 5g **Sodium:** 30mg

Ingredients:

2 chicken breasts (about 6 ounces each)

A pinch of salt and pepper

2 potatoes, peeled and cubed

1/4 cup milk (or dairy-free alternative)

1 tablespoon butter (or olive oil)

1 cup carrots, sliced

Method of Preparation:

1. Preheat the oven to 375°F (190°C).
2. Season the chicken breasts with salt and pepper on both sides.
3. Place the seasoned chicken breasts on a baking sheet lined with parchment paper.
4. Bake in the preheated oven for 25-30 minutes, or until the chicken is cooked through and no longer pink in the center.
5. While the chicken is baking, cook the cubed potatoes in boiling water until tender, about 15 minutes.
6. Drain the cooked potatoes and transfer them to a mixing bowl.
7. Add milk and butter to the potatoes and mash until smooth and creamy. Season with salt and pepper to taste.
8. Steam sliced carrots until tender, about 5-7 minutes.

9. Serve the baked chicken breast with mashed potatoes and steamed carrots.

Poached Salmon with White Rice and Cooked Spinach

Preparation time: 20 minutes

Serves: 2

Calories: 400 **Carbs:** 40g **Protein:** 30g **Fat:** 15g **Fiber:** 3g **Sodium:** 100mg

Ingredients:

2 salmon fillets (about 6 ounces each)

A pinch of salt and pepper

1 cup white rice, cooked

2 cups spinach leaves

Lemon wedges (optional, for serving)

Method of Preparation:

1. Season the salmon fillets with salt and pepper on both sides.

2. In a large skillet, bring about 2 cups of water to a simmer over medium heat.
3. Gently add the seasoned salmon fillets to the simmering water.
4. Cover the skillet and poach the salmon for 8-10 minutes, or until the salmon is cooked through and flakes easily with a fork.
5. While the salmon is poaching, cook white rice according to package instructions.
6. In a separate skillet, wilt spinach leaves over medium heat for 2-3 minutes.
7. Serve the poached salmon with cooked white rice and wilted spinach. Garnish with lemon wedges if desired.

HIGH FIBER DIET

BREAKFAST

Whole Grain Toast with Avocado and Poached Eggs

Preparation time: 15 minutes

Serves: 2

Calories: 300 **Carbs:** 25g **Protein:** 12g **Fat:** 18g **Fiber:** 10g **Sodium:** 30mg

Ingredients:

2 slices whole grain bread, toasted

1 ripe avocado, mashed

2 eggs

A pinch of salt and pepper

Lemon juice (optional, for serving)

Red pepper flakes (optional, for serving)

Fresh herbs (such as cilantro or parsley), chopped (optional, for garnish)

Method of Preparation:

1. Poach the eggs
2. Fill a saucepan with water and bring it to a gentle simmer over medium heat.
3. Crack one egg into a small bowl or ramekin.
4. Carefully slide the egg into the simmering water.
5. Repeat with the second egg.

6. Poach the eggs for 3-4 minutes until the whites are set but the yolks are still runny.
7. Use a slotted spoon to remove the poached eggs from the water and drain excess water.
8. Spread mashed avocado evenly over the toasted whole grain bread slices.
9. Place one poached egg on top of each avocado-covered toast.
10. Season with salt and pepper to taste. Optionally, drizzle with lemon juice and sprinkle with red pepper flakes for extra flavor.
11. Garnish with chopped fresh herbs if desired and serve immediately.

Greek Yogurt Parfait with Berries and Granola

Preparation time: 5 minutes

Serves: 2

Calories: 250 **Carbs:** 30g **Protein:** 15g **Fat:** 8g **Fiber:** 5g **Sodium:** 50mg

Ingredients:

1 cup Greek yogurt (unsweetened)

1/2 cup mixed berries (such as strawberries, blueberries, and raspberries)

1/4 cup granola (low sugar)

Honey or maple syrup (optional, for sweetness)

Method of Preparation:

1. In two serving glasses or bowls, layer Greek yogurt, mixed berries, and granola.
2. If desired, drizzle honey or maple syrup over the layers for added sweetness.
3. Repeat layering until all ingredients are used up.
4. Serve immediately as a parfait.

Whole Grain Pancakes Topped with Greek Yogurt and Mixed Berries

Preparation time: 15 minutes

Serves: 2

Calories: 300 **Carbs:** 40g **Protein:** 15g **Fat:** 8g **Fiber:** 5g **Sodium:** 40mg

Ingredients:

1 cup whole grain pancake mix

1/2 cup water (or as needed to reach desired consistency)

1/2 cup Greek yogurt (unsweetened)

1/2 cup mixed berries (such as strawberries, blueberries, and raspberries)

Honey or maple syrup (optional, for sweetness)

Method of Preparation:

1. In a mixing bowl, prepare the pancake batter according to package instructions by combining whole grain pancake mix and water.
2. Heat a non-stick skillet or griddle over medium heat. Pour pancake batter onto the skillet to form pancakes of desired size.
3. Cook pancakes until bubbles form on the surface, then flip and cook until golden brown on both sides.

4. Serve pancakes topped with Greek yogurt and mixed berries.
5. Optionally, drizzle with honey or maple syrup for added sweetness.
6. Serve immediately.

Quinoa Breakfast Bowl with Sautéed Vegetables and a Poached Egg

Preparation time: 30 minutes

Serves: 2

Calories: 300 **Carbs:** 25g **Protein:** 15g **Fat:** 15g **Fiber:** 5g **Sodium:** 150mg

Ingredients:

1/2 cup quinoa, rinsed

1 cup water or vegetable broth (low sodium)

1 tablespoon olive oil

1/2 cup mixed vegetables (such as bell peppers, onions, and spinach), chopped

2 eggs

A pinch of salt and pepper

Fresh herbs (such as parsley or chives), chopped (optional, for garnish)

Method of Preparation:

1. In a saucepan, combine quinoa and water or vegetable broth. Bring to a boil, then reduce heat to low, cover, and simmer for 15-20 minutes until quinoa is cooked and liquid is absorbed.
2. While quinoa is cooking, heat olive oil in a skillet over medium heat. Add chopped mixed vegetables and sauté until tender, about 5-7 minutes.
3. In a separate saucepan, poach the eggs: Fill the saucepan with water and bring it to a gentle simmer. Crack one egg into a small bowl or ramekin. Carefully slide the egg into the simmering water. Repeat with the second egg. Poach the eggs for 3-4 minutes until the whites are set but the yolks are still runny. Use a slotted spoon to remove the poached eggs from the water and drain excess water.

4. To assemble the breakfast bowl, divide cooked quinoa among two bowls. Top with sautéed vegetables and a poached egg.
5. Season with salt and pepper to taste. Garnish with chopped fresh herbs if desired and serve immediately.

Whole Grain Muffins with Mashed Sweet Potato and Pecans

Preparation time: 30 minutes

Serves: 2

Calories: 300 **Carbs:** 40g **Protein:** 5g **Fat:** 10g **Fiber:** 5g **Sodium:** 50mg

Ingredients:

1 cup whole wheat flour

1 teaspoon baking powder

1/2 teaspoon baking soda

1/4 teaspoon salt

1/2 cup mashed sweet potato

1/4 cup maple syrup

1/4 cup milk (or dairy-free alternative)

1/4 cup chopped pecans

Method of Preparation:

1. Preheat the oven to 350°F (175°C). Line a muffin tin with paper liners or lightly grease with oil.
2. In a mixing bowl, combine whole wheat flour, baking powder, baking soda, and salt.
3. In another bowl, mix together mashed sweet potato, maple syrup, and milk until well combined.
4. Add the wet ingredients to the dry ingredients and stir until just combined. Fold in chopped pecans.
5. Divide the batter evenly among the prepared muffin cups.
6. Bake in the preheated oven for 18-20 minutes, or until a toothpick inserted into the center comes out clean.
7. Remove muffins from the oven and let them cool in the pan for a few minutes before transferring to a wire rack to cool completely.
8. Serve warm or at room temperature.

Chia Seed Pudding Topped with Sliced Almonds and Fresh Fruit

Preparation time: 5 minutes (plus chilling time)

Serves: 2

Calories: 200 **Carbs:** 20g **Protein:** 5g **Fat:** 10g **Fiber:** 10g **Sodium:** 50mg

Ingredients:

1/4 cup chia seeds

1 cup milk (or dairy-free alternative)

1 tablespoon honey or maple syrup (optional, for sweetness)

Sliced almonds, for topping

Fresh fruit (such as berries, sliced banana, or diced mango), for topping

Method of Preparation:

1. In a mixing bowl, combine chia seeds, milk, and honey or maple syrup (if using). Stir well to combine.

2. Cover the bowl and refrigerate for at least 2 hours or overnight, until the mixture thickens and becomes pudding-like.
3. Once the chia seed pudding has set, divide it into two serving bowls.
4. Top each bowl of chia seed pudding with sliced almonds and fresh fruit.
5. Serve chilled.

Whole Grain Waffles with Almond Butter and Sliced Strawberries

Preparation time: 5 minutes

Serves: 2

Calories: 300 **Carbs:** 35g **Protein:** 8g **Fat:** 15g **Fiber:** 7g **Sodium:** 150mg

Ingredients:

2 whole grain waffles (store-bought or homemade)

2 tablespoons almond butter

1/2 cup sliced strawberries

Method of Preparation:

1. Toast the whole grain waffles until golden brown and crispy.
2. Spread almond butter evenly over each toasted waffle.
3. Arrange sliced strawberries on top of the almond butter.
4. Serve immediately.

Breakfast Burrito filled with Scrambled Eggs, Black Beans, Avocado, and Salsa

Preparation time: 15 minutes

Serves: 2

Calories: 400 **Carbs:** 40g **Protein:** 18g **Fat:** 20g **Fiber:** 12g **Sodium:** 60mg

Ingredients:

2 large whole grain tortillas

4 eggs, scrambled

1/2 cup black beans, cooked and drained

1 avocado, sliced

1/4 cup salsa

A pinch of salt and pepper

Method of Preparation:

1. Warm the whole grain tortillas in a dry skillet or microwave for a few seconds until soft and pliable.
2. Divide scrambled eggs, black beans, avocado slices, and salsa evenly between the two tortillas.
3. Season with salt and pepper to taste.
4. Fold the sides of each tortilla inward, then roll up tightly to form a burrito.
5. Serve immediately.

LUNCH

Quinoa Salad with Chickpeas and Mixed Vegetables

Preparation time: 25 minutes

Serves: 2

Calories: 400 **Carbs:** 55g **Protein:** 15g **Fat:** 15g **Fiber:** 10g **Sodium:** 30mg

Ingredients:

1 cup quinoa, rinsed

2 cups water or vegetable broth (low sodium)

1 can (15 ounces) chickpeas, drained and rinsed

1 cup mixed vegetables (such as bell peppers, cucumbers, cherry tomatoes), diced

1/4 cup fresh parsley, chopped

2 tablespoons olive oil

1 tablespoon lemon juice

A pinch of salt and pepper

Method of Preparation:

1. In a saucepan, combine quinoa and water or vegetable broth. Bring to a boil, then reduce heat to low, cover, and simmer for 15-20 minutes until quinoa is cooked and liquid is absorbed.

2. Fluff the cooked quinoa with a fork and transfer it to a large mixing bowl.
3. Add chickpeas, mixed vegetables, and chopped parsley to the bowl with quinoa.
4. In a small bowl, whisk together olive oil, lemon juice, salt, and pepper to make the dressing.
5. Pour the dressing over the quinoa salad and toss until well combined.
6. Serve immediately or refrigerate for later.

Lentil Soup with Spinach and Tomatoes

Preparation time: 40 minutes

Serves: 2

Calories: 350 **Carbs:** 55g **Protein:** 20g **Fat:** 5g **Fiber:** 20g **Sodium:** 60mg

Ingredients:

1 cup dried lentils, rinsed

4 cups vegetable broth (low sodium)

1 onion, chopped

2 cloves garlic, minced

1 can (14 ounces) diced tomatoes

2 cups fresh spinach leaves

1 teaspoon dried thyme

A pinch of salt and pepper

Method of Preparation:

1. In a large pot, combine dried lentils and vegetable broth. Bring to a boil, then reduce heat to low, cover, and simmer for 20-25 minutes until lentils are tender.
2. In a skillet, heat olive oil over medium heat. Add chopped onion and minced garlic. Cook until onions are translucent.
3. Add diced tomatoes (with juices) to the skillet and cook for 5 minutes.
4. Add the cooked lentils and vegetable broth to the skillet. Stir in fresh spinach leaves and dried thyme.
5. Season with salt and pepper to taste. Simmer for an additional 5-10 minutes until spinach is wilted.
6. Serve hot.

Grilled Chicken and Vegetable Wrap with Whole Grain Tortilla

Preparation time: 20 minutes

Serves: 2

Calories: 450 **Carbs:** 40g **Protein:** 30g **Fat:** 20g **Fiber:** 8g **Sodium:** 80mg

Ingredients:

2 boneless, skinless chicken breasts

A pinch of salt and pepper

2 whole grain tortillas

1 cup mixed vegetables (such as bell peppers, zucchini, onions), sliced

2 tablespoons olive oil

1/4 cup Greek yogurt (unsweetened)

2 tablespoons hummus (optional)

Method of Preparation:

1. Season chicken breasts with salt and pepper.

2. Grill or cook in a skillet until cooked through, about 6-8 minutes per side.
3. Slice cooked chicken into strips.
4. In a skillet, heat olive oil over medium heat.
5. Add mixed vegetables and cook until tender, about 5-7 minutes.
6. Warm whole grain tortillas in a dry skillet or microwave for a few seconds until soft.
7. Spread Greek yogurt and hummus (if using) evenly over each tortilla.
8. Arrange sliced grilled chicken and cooked mixed vegetables on top of the tortillas.
9. Roll up the tortillas tightly to form wraps.
10. Serve immediately or wrap in foil for later.

Brown Rice Stir-Fry with Tofu and Broccoli

Preparation time: 50 minutes

Serves: 2

Calories: 400 **Carbs:** 50g **Protein:** 20g **Fat:** 15g **Fiber:** 8g **Sodium:** 50mg

Ingredients:

1 cup brown rice

2 cups water

1 tablespoon olive oil

1 block (14 ounces) firm tofu, cubed

2 cups broccoli florets

1 bell pepper, sliced

1 carrot, julienned

2 cloves garlic, minced

2 tablespoons soy sauce (low sodium)

1 tablespoon sesame oil

Sesame seeds, for garnish (optional)

Method of Preparation:

1. In a saucepan, combine brown rice and water. Bring to a boil, then reduce heat to low, cover, and simmer for 40-45 minutes until rice is cooked and water is absorbed.

2. While the rice is cooking, heat olive oil in a large skillet or wok over medium-high heat. Add cubed tofu and cook until golden brown on all sides. Remove tofu from the skillet and set aside.
3. In the same skillet, add broccoli florets, sliced bell pepper, julienned carrot, and minced garlic. Stir-fry for 5-7 minutes until vegetables are tender-crisp.
4. Return cooked tofu to the skillet and add cooked brown rice.
5. Drizzle soy sauce and sesame oil over the stir-fry. Toss everything together until well combined and heated through.
6. Garnish with sesame seeds if desired and serve hot.

Turkey and Black Bean Chili with Whole Grain Cornbread

Preparation time: 1 hour

Serves: 2

Calories: 350 **Carbs:** 30g **Protein:** 25g **Fat:** 15g **Fiber:** 10g **Sodium:** 90mg

Ingredients for Chili:

1 tablespoon olive oil

1 onion, chopped

2 cloves garlic, minced

1 pound ground turkey

1 can (14 ounces) diced tomatoes

1 can (14 ounces) black beans, drained and rinsed

1 cup vegetable broth (low sodium)

1 tablespoon chili powder

1 teaspoon ground cumin

A pinch of salt and pepper

Ingredients for Cornbread:

1 cup whole grain cornmeal

1/2 cup whole wheat flour

1 tablespoon baking powder

1/4 teaspoon salt

1/4 cup honey or maple syrup

1/4 cup unsweetened applesauce

1/2 cup milk (or dairy-free alternative)

1 egg

Method of Preparation:

1. In a large pot, heat olive oil over medium heat.
2. Add chopped onion and minced garlic.
3. Cook until onions are translucent.
4. Add ground turkey to the pot and cook until browned, breaking it up with a spoon.
5. Stir in diced tomatoes, black beans, vegetable broth, chili powder, and ground cumin.
6. Season with salt and pepper to taste.
7. Bring the chili to a simmer, then reduce heat to low.
8. Cover and cook for 20-30 minutes, stirring occasionally.
9. While the chili is cooking, preheat the oven to 400°F (200°C).
10. Grease a baking dish or line with parchment paper.
11. In a mixing bowl, combine whole grain cornmeal, whole wheat flour, baking powder, and salt.

12. In another bowl, whisk together honey or maple syrup, unsweetened applesauce, milk, and egg.
13. Pour the wet ingredients into the dry ingredients and stir until just combined.
14. Pour the cornbread batter into the prepared baking dish and spread evenly.
15. Bake in the preheated oven for 20-25 minutes, or until a toothpick inserted into the center comes out clean.
16. Serve the turkey and black bean chili with whole grain cornbread.

Greek Salad with Mixed Greens, Cucumber, Tomato, Feta, and Chickpeas

Preparation time: 10 minutes

Serves: 2

Calories: 350 **Carbs:** 30g **Protein:** 12g **Fat:** 20g **Fiber:** 8g **Sodium:** 100mg

Ingredients:

4 cups mixed greens (such as lettuce, spinach, and arugula)

1 cucumber, diced

2 tomatoes, diced

1/2 cup feta cheese, crumbled

1 can (15 ounces) chickpeas, drained and rinsed

2 tablespoons extra virgin olive oil

1 tablespoon red wine vinegar

1 teaspoon dried oregano

A pinch of salt and pepper

Method of Preparation:

1. In a large salad bowl, combine mixed greens, diced cucumber, diced tomatoes, crumbled feta cheese, and drained chickpeas.
2. In a small bowl, whisk together extra virgin olive oil, red wine vinegar, dried oregano, salt, and pepper to make the dressing.

3. Pour the dressing over the salad and toss until well combined.
4. Serve immediately.

Whole Wheat Pasta Primavera with Grilled Shrimp

Preparation time: 30 minutes

Serves: 2

Calories: 400 **Carbs:** 50g **Protein:** 25g **Fat:** 10g **Fiber:** 10g **Sodium:** 100mg

Ingredients:

8 ounces whole wheat pasta

1 tablespoon olive oil

1 onion, diced

2 cloves garlic, minced

2 cups mixed vegetables (such as bell peppers, zucchini, and cherry tomatoes), sliced

1/2-pound shrimp, peeled and deveined

A pinch of salt and pepper

1/4 cup grated Parmesan cheese (optional, for serving)

Fresh basil leaves, chopped (optional, for garnish)

Method of Preparation:

1. Cook whole wheat pasta according to package instructions until al dente.
2. Drain and set aside.
3. In a large skillet, heat olive oil over medium heat.
4. Add diced onion and minced garlic.
5. Cook until onions are translucent.
6. Add sliced mixed vegetables to the skillet and cook until tender-crisp, about 5-7 minutes.
7. Season shrimp with salt and pepper.
8. Add shrimp to the skillet and cook until pink and opaque, about 2-3 minutes per side.
9. Add cooked whole wheat pasta to the skillet with the vegetables and shrimp.
10. Toss everything together until well combined.
11. Serve pasta primavera hot, optionally topped with grated Parmesan cheese and chopped fresh basil.

DINNER

Roasted Vegetable and Barley Pilaf

Preparation time: 50 minutes

Serves: 2

Calories: 350 **Carbs:** 60g **Protein:** 8g **Fat:** 8g **Fiber:** 12g **Sodium:** 40mg

Ingredients:

1 cup barley

2 cups vegetable broth (low sodium)

2 cups mixed vegetables (such as bell peppers, zucchini, carrots), diced

1 onion, chopped

2 cloves garlic, minced

2 tablespoons olive oil

A pinch of salt and pepper

Fresh parsley, chopped (optional, for garnish)

Method of Preparation:

1. Preheat the oven to 400°F (200°C).
2. In a saucepan, combine barley and vegetable broth.
3. Bring to a boil, then reduce heat to low, cover, and simmer for 30-40 minutes until barley is tender and liquid is absorbed.
4. While the barley is cooking, spread diced mixed vegetables, chopped onion, and minced garlic on a baking sheet.
5. Drizzle with olive oil and season with salt and pepper.
6. Toss to coat evenly.
7. Roast vegetables in the preheated oven for 20-25 minutes, or until tender and lightly browned.
8. Once the barley and vegetables are cooked, combine them in a large mixing bowl.
9. Toss until well combined.
10. Serve the roasted vegetable and barley pilaf hot, optionally garnished with chopped fresh parsley.

Bean and Vegetable Burrito Bowls

Preparation time: 50 minutes

Serves: 2

Calories: 400 **Carbs:** 65g **Protein:** 12g **Fat:** 10g **Fiber:** 15g **Sodium:** 80mg

Ingredients:

1 cup brown rice

2 cups water

1 can (15 ounces) black beans, drained and rinsed

1 cup corn kernels (fresh or frozen)

1 bell pepper, diced

1 avocado, sliced

1/4 cup salsa

1/4 cup Greek yogurt (unsweetened)

Fresh cilantro, chopped (optional, for garnish)

Method of Preparation:

1. In a saucepan, combine brown rice and water.

2. Bring to a boil, then reduce heat to low, cover, and simmer for 40-45 minutes until rice is cooked and water is absorbed.
3. While the rice is cooking, prepare the black beans, corn kernels, diced bell pepper, and sliced avocado.
4. Once the rice is cooked, divide it into two serving bowls.
5. Top each bowl with black beans, corn kernels, diced bell pepper, sliced avocado, salsa, and Greek yogurt.
6. Garnish with chopped fresh cilantro if desired.
7. Serve the bean and vegetable burrito bowls hot.

Spinach and Feta Stuffed Chicken Breast with Quinoa Pilaf

Preparation time: 40 minutes

Serves: 2

Calories: 350 **Carbs:** 20g **Protein:** 30g **Fat:** 15g **Fiber:** 5g **Sodium:** 100mg

Ingredients:

2 boneless, skinless chicken breasts

A pinch of salt and pepper

1 cup cooked quinoa

1 cup spinach leaves, chopped

1/4 cup feta cheese, crumbled

1 tablespoon olive oil

1 lemon, sliced (optional, for serving)

Fresh parsley, chopped (optional, for garnish)

Method of Preparation:

1. Preheat the oven to 375°F (190°C).
2. Cut a slit horizontally through the thickest part of each chicken breast to create a pocket.
3. Season the chicken breasts with salt and pepper, both inside and out.
4. In a mixing bowl, combine cooked quinoa, chopped spinach leaves, and crumbled feta cheese. Mix until well combined.
5. Stuff each chicken breast with the quinoa-spinach-feta mixture, pressing gently to seal the openings.

6. Heat olive oil in an oven-safe skillet over medium-high heat. Add stuffed chicken breasts to the skillet and sear for 2-3 minutes on each side until golden brown.
7. Transfer the skillet to the preheated oven and bake for 20-25 minutes until the chicken is cooked through and no longer pink in the center.
8. Serve the spinach and feta stuffed chicken breast hot, optionally garnished with lemon slices and chopped fresh parsley.

Lentil Soup with Whole Grain Bread

Preparation time: 40 minutes

Serves: 2

Calories: 350 **Carbs:** 60g **Protein:** 20g **Fat:** 5g **Fiber:** 20g **Sodium:** 60mg

Ingredients:

1 cup dried lentils, rinsed

4 cups vegetable broth (low sodium)

1 onion, chopped

2 carrots, diced

2 celery stalks, diced

2 cloves garlic, minced

1 can (14 ounces) diced tomatoes

1 teaspoon ground cumin

1 teaspoon ground coriander

A pinch of salt and pepper

Fresh parsley, chopped (optional, for garnish)

Whole grain bread, sliced (for serving)

Method of Preparation:

1. In a large pot, combine dried lentils and vegetable broth.
2. Bring to a boil, then reduce heat to low, cover, and simmer for 20-25 minutes until lentils are tender.
3. In the meantime, heat olive oil in a skillet over medium heat.
4. Add chopped onion, diced carrots, diced celery, and minced garlic.
5. Cook until vegetables are tender, about 5-7 minutes.

6. Add diced tomatoes (with juices), ground cumin, and ground coriander to the skillet.
7. Cook for an additional 5 minutes.
8. Once the lentils are cooked, add the cooked vegetable mixture to the pot with the lentils and broth. Stir to combine.
9. Season with salt and pepper to taste.
10. Simmer for an additional 10-15 minutes to allow flavors to meld.
11. Serve the lentil soup hot, garnished with chopped fresh parsley.
12. Serve with sliced whole grain bread on the side.

Chickpea Curry with Brown Rice

Preparation time: 45 minutes

Serves: 2

Calories: 400 **Carbs:** 60g **Protein:** 15g **Fat:** 12g **Fiber:** 10g **Sodium:** 90mg

Ingredients:

1 cup brown rice

2 cups water

1 tablespoon olive oil

1 onion, chopped

2 cloves garlic, minced

1 can (15 ounces) chickpeas, drained and rinsed

1 can (14 ounces) diced tomatoes

1 can (14 ounces) coconut milk (full fat or light)

2 tablespoons curry powder

A pinch of salt and pepper

Fresh cilantro, chopped (optional, for garnish)

Method of Preparation:

1. In a saucepan, combine brown rice and water.
2. Bring to a boil, then reduce heat to low, cover, and simmer for 40-45 minutes until rice is cooked and water is absorbed.
3. While the rice is cooking, heat olive oil in a large skillet over medium heat.
4. Add chopped onion and minced garlic.
5. Cook until onions are translucent.

6. Add drained chickpeas, diced tomatoes (with juices), coconut milk, and curry powder to the skillet.
7. Stir to combine.
8. Bring the mixture to a simmer and cook for 15-20 minutes, stirring occasionally, until the flavors meld and the sauce thickens.
9. Season with salt and pepper to taste.
10. Serve the chickpea curry hot, spooned over cooked brown rice.
11. Garnish with chopped fresh cilantro if desired.

Turkey and Black Bean Chili with Cornbread

Preparation time: 1 hour

Serves: 2

Calories: 350 **Carbs:** 30g **Protein:** 25g **Fat:** 15g **Fiber:** 10g **Sodium:** 100mg

Ingredients for Chili:

1 tablespoon olive oil

1 onion, diced

2 cloves garlic, minced

1 pound ground turkey

1 can (14 ounces) diced tomatoes

1 can (14 ounces) black beans, drained and rinsed

1 cup vegetable broth (low sodium)

1 tablespoon chili powder

1 teaspoon ground cumin

A pinch of salt and pepper

Ingredients for Cornbread:

1 cup whole grain cornmeal

1/2 cup whole wheat flour

1 tablespoon baking powder

1/4 teaspoon salt

1/4 cup honey or maple syrup

1/4 cup unsweetened applesauce

1/2 cup milk (or dairy-free alternative)

1 egg

Method of Preparation:

1. In a large pot, heat olive oil over medium heat.
2. Add diced onion and minced garlic.
3. Cook until onions are translucent.
4. Add ground turkey to the pot and cook until browned, breaking it up with a spoon.
5. Stir in diced tomatoes, black beans, vegetable broth, chili powder, and ground cumin.
6. Season with salt and pepper to taste.
7. Bring the chili to a simmer, then reduce heat to low.
8. Cover and cook for 20-30 minutes, stirring occasionally.
9. While the chili is cooking, preheat the oven to 400°F (200°C).
10. Grease a baking dish or line with parchment paper.
11. In a mixing bowl, combine whole grain cornmeal, whole wheat flour, baking powder, and salt.
12. In another bowl, whisk together honey or maple syrup, unsweetened applesauce, milk, and egg.
13. Pour the wet ingredients into the dry ingredients and stir until just combined.

14. Pour the cornbread batter into the prepared baking dish and spread evenly.
15. Bake in the preheated oven for 20-25 minutes, or until a toothpick inserted into the center comes out clean.
16. Serve the turkey and black bean chili with slices of cornbread.

Grilled Chicken Salad with Mixed Greens, Avocado, and Beans

Preparation time: 20 minutes

Serves: 2

Calories: 400 **Carbs:** 30g **Protein:** 30g **Fat:** 20g **Fiber:** 12g **Sodium:** 50mg

Ingredients:

2 boneless, skinless chicken breasts

A pinch of salt and pepper

4 cups mixed greens (such as lettuce, spinach, and arugula)

1 avocado, sliced

1 can (15 ounces) beans (such as black beans or chickpeas), drained and rinsed

1/4 cup balsamic vinaigrette dressing (low sodium)

Method of Preparation:

1. Preheat the grill to medium-high heat.
2. Season chicken breasts with salt and pepper.
3. Grill chicken breasts for 6-8 minutes per side, or until cooked through and no longer pink in the center. Remove from grill and let them rest for a few minutes before slicing.
4. In a large salad bowl, combine mixed greens, sliced avocado, and drained beans.
5. Slice grilled chicken breasts and add them to the salad bowl.
6. Drizzle balsamic vinaigrette dressing over the salad and toss until well combined.
7. Serve the grilled chicken salad immediately.

DESSERTS

Fruit Salad with Melons, Berries, and a Squeeze of Lime Juice

Preparation time: 10 minutes

Serves: 2

Calories: 100 **Carbs:** 25g **Protein:** 2g **Fat:** 0g **Fiber:** 5g **Sodium:** 10mg

Ingredients:

1 cup diced cantaloupe

1 cup diced honeydew melon

1 cup mixed berries (such as strawberries, blueberries, raspberries)

1 lime, juiced

Method of Preparation:

1. In a large mixing bowl, combine diced cantaloupe, diced honeydew melon, and mixed berries.
2. Squeeze lime juice over the fruit salad.

3. Toss gently until the fruit is evenly coated with lime juice.
4. Serve the fruit salad immediately or refrigerate until ready to serve.

Banana Oatmeal Cookies made with Mashed Bananas and Oats

Preparation time: 25 minutes

Serves: 2

Calories: 150 **Carbs:** 30g **Protein:** 3g **Fat:** 2g **Fiber:** 4g **Sodium:** 0mg

Ingredients:

2 ripe bananas, mashed

1 cup rolled oats

1/4 cup raisins or dried cranberries (optional)

1/4 teaspoon cinnamon

1/4 teaspoon vanilla extract (optional)

Method of Preparation:

1. Preheat the oven to 350°F (175°C).
2. Line a baking sheet with parchment paper.
3. In a mixing bowl, combine mashed bananas, rolled oats, raisins or dried cranberries (if using), cinnamon, and vanilla extract (if using).
4. Mix until well combined.
5. Drop spoonful of the cookie dough onto the prepared baking sheet, spacing them apart.
6. Flatten each cookie slightly with the back of a spoon.
7. Bake in the preheated oven for 15-20 minutes, or until the cookies are golden brown and set.
8. Remove from the oven and let the cookies cool on the baking sheet for a few minutes before transferring them to a wire rack to cool completely.

Baked Apples with Cinnamon and a Sprinkle of Oats

Preparation time: 30 minutes

Serves: 2

Calories: 150 **Carbs:** 35g **Protein:** 2g **Fat:** 1g **Fiber:** 6g **Sodium:** 0mg

Ingredients:

2 apples

1 teaspoon ground cinnamon

2 tablespoons rolled oats

1 tablespoon honey (optional)

Method of Preparation:

1. Preheat the oven to 375°F (190°C).
2. Line a baking dish with parchment paper.
3. Core the apples and cut them in half horizontally.
4. Place the apple halves cut-side up in the prepared baking dish.
5. Sprinkle ground cinnamon evenly over the apple halves.
6. Top each apple half with rolled oats.
7. Drizzle honey over the apples, if using.
8. Bake in the preheated oven for 20-25 minutes, or until the apples are tender.
9. Serve the baked apples warm.

Greek Yogurt with Honey and Sliced Strawberries

Preparation time: 5 minutes

Serves: 2

Calories: 150 **Carbs:** 20g **Protein:** 12g **Fat:** 3g **Fiber:** 2g **Sodium:** 50mg

Ingredients:

1 cup Greek yogurt (unsweetened)

1 tablespoon honey

1/2 cup sliced strawberries

Method of Preparation:

1. In a serving bowl, spoon Greek yogurt.
2. Drizzle honey over the yogurt.
3. Arrange sliced strawberries on top of the yogurt.
4. Serve the Greek yogurt with honey and sliced strawberries immediately.

Poached Pears with a Drizzle of Dark Chocolate Sauce

Preparation time: 25 minutes

Serves: 2

Calories: 200 **Carbs:** 50g **Protein:** 1g **Fat:** 1g **Fiber:** 6g **Sodium:** 0mg

Ingredients:

2 ripe pears

2 cups water

1/4 cup honey

1 teaspoon vanilla extract

Dark chocolate sauce (store-bought or homemade)

Method of Preparation:

1. Peel the pears, leaving the stems intact. Cut a thin slice off the bottom of each pear to create a flat base for stability.
2. In a pot, combine water, honey, and vanilla extract. Bring to a simmer over medium heat.

3. Add the pears to the pot, ensuring they are submerged in the liquid. Simmer gently for 15-20 minutes, or until the pears are tender when pierced with a knife.
4. Remove the pears from the pot and let them cool slightly.
5. Serve the poached pears with a drizzle of dark chocolate sauce.

SOUPS AND STEWS

Lentil Stew

Preparation time: 45 minutes

Serves: 2

Calories: 300 **Carbs:** 50g **Protein:** 18g **Fat:** 2g **Fiber:** 18g **Sodium:** 100mg

Ingredients:

1 cup dried lentils, rinsed

4 cups vegetable broth (low sodium)

1 onion, chopped

2 carrots, diced

2 celery stalks, diced

2 cloves garlic, minced

1 can (14 ounces) diced tomatoes

1 teaspoon dried thyme

1 teaspoon dried rosemary

A pinch of salt and pepper

Method of Preparation:

1. In a large pot, combine dried lentils and vegetable broth.
2. Bring to a boil, then reduce heat to low, cover, and simmer for 20-25 minutes until lentils are tender.
3. In the meantime, heat olive oil in a skillet over medium heat.
4. Add chopped onion, diced carrots, diced celery, and minced garlic.
5. Cook until vegetables are tender, about 5-7 minutes.
6. Add diced tomatoes (with juices), dried thyme, and dried rosemary to the skillet.

7. Cook for an additional 5 minutes.
8. Once the lentils are cooked, add the cooked vegetable mixture to the pot with the lentils and broth.
9. Stir to combine.
10. Season with salt and pepper to taste.
11. Simmer for an additional 10-15 minutes to allow flavors to meld.
12. Serve the lentil stew hot.

Turkey Chili

Preparation time: 30 minutes

Serves: 2

Calories: 350 **Carbs:** 30g **Protein:** 30g **Fat:** 10g **Fiber:** 10g **Sodium:** 50mg

Ingredients:

1 tablespoon olive oil

1 onion, diced

2 cloves garlic, minced

1 pound ground turkey

1 can (14 ounces) diced tomatoes

1 can (14 ounces) kidney beans, drained and rinsed

1 cup vegetable broth (low sodium)

1 tablespoon chili powder

1 teaspoon ground cumin

A pinch of salt and pepper

Method of Preparation:

1. In a large pot, heat olive oil over medium heat.
2. Add diced onion and minced garlic.
3. Cook until onions are translucent.
4. Add ground turkey to the pot and cook until browned, breaking it up with a spoon.
5. Stir in diced tomatoes, kidney beans, vegetable broth, chili powder, and ground cumin. Season with salt and pepper to taste.
6. Bring the chili to a simmer, then reduce heat to low.
7. Cover and cook for 20-30 minutes, stirring occasionally.
8. Serve the turkey chili hot.

Minestrone Soup

Preparation time: 40 minutes

Serves: 2

Calories: 300 **Carbs:** 50g **Protein:** 15g **Fat:** 5g **Fiber:** 10g **Sodium:** 100mg

Ingredients:

1 tablespoon olive oil

1 onion, diced

2 cloves garlic, minced

2 carrots, diced

2 celery stalks, diced

1 zucchini, diced

1 can (14 ounces) diced tomatoes

4 cups vegetable broth (low sodium)

1 can (14 ounces) kidney beans, drained and rinsed

1/2 cup whole grain pasta

1 teaspoon dried oregano

1 teaspoon dried basil

A pinch of salt and pepper

Method of Preparation:

1. In a large pot, heat olive oil over medium heat.
2. Add diced onion and minced garlic.
3. Cook until onions are translucent.
4. Add diced carrots, diced celery, and diced zucchini to the pot.
5. Cook for 5-7 minutes until vegetables are tender.
6. Stir in diced tomatoes, vegetable broth, kidney beans, whole grain pasta, dried oregano, and dried basil.
7. Season with salt and pepper to taste.
8. Bring the soup to a boil, then reduce heat to low.
9. Cover and simmer for 15-20 minutes, or until pasta is cooked and vegetables are tender.
10. Serve the minestrone soup hot.

Split Pea Soup

Preparation time: 1 hour

Serves: 2

Calories: 250 **Carbs:** 45g **Protein:** 15g **Fat:** 1g **Fiber:** 20g **Sodium:** 50mg

Ingredients:

1 cup dried split peas, rinsed

4 cups vegetable broth (low sodium)

1 onion, chopped

2 carrots, diced

2 celery stalks, diced

2 cloves garlic, minced

1 bay leaf

A pinch of salt and pepper

Method of Preparation:

1. In a large pot, combine dried split peas and vegetable broth.
2. Bring to a boil, then reduce heat to low, cover, and simmer for 40-45 minutes until peas are tender.

3. In the meantime, heat olive oil in a skillet over medium heat.
4. Add chopped onion, diced carrots, diced celery, and minced garlic.
5. Cook until vegetables are tender, about 5-7 minutes.
6. Add the cooked vegetables to the pot with the split peas.
7. Add a bay leaf to the pot and season with salt and pepper to taste.
8. Simmer the soup for an additional 10-15 minutes to allow flavors to meld.
9. Serve the split pea soup hot.

Beef and Barley Stew

Preparation time: 1.5 hours

Serves: 2

Calories: 400 **Carbs:** 45g **Protein:** 25g **Fat:** 10g **Fiber:** 8g **Sodium:** 60mg

Ingredients:

½-pound beef stew meat, cubed

1 tablespoon olive oil

1 onion, chopped

2 carrots, diced

2 celery stalks, diced

2 cloves garlic, minced

4 cups beef broth (low sodium)

1/2 cup pearl barley

1 bay leaf

A pinch of salt and pepper

Method of Preparation:

1. In a large pot, heat olive oil over medium heat.
2. Add cubed beef stew meat and cook until browned on all sides.
3. Remove from the pot and set aside.
4. In the same pot, add chopped onion, diced carrots, diced celery, and minced garlic.
5. Cook until vegetables are tender, about 5-7 minutes.
6. Return the browned beef to the pot.
7. Add beef broth, pearl barley, and a bay leaf.
8. Season with salt and pepper to taste.
9. Bring the stew to a boil, then reduce heat to low.
10. Cover and simmer for 1-1.5 hours, or until beef is tender and barley is cooked.
11. Remove the bay leaf before serving.
12. Serve the beef and barley stew hot.

CONCLUSION

In conclusion, managing diverticulitis effectively involves a multifaceted approach that encompasses dietary modifications, lifestyle changes, and medical treatment when necessary.

By adhering to a diet high in fiber and fluids, individuals with diverticulitis can promote bowel regularity, reduce inflammation, and alleviate symptoms.

Additionally, avoiding foods that may exacerbate symptoms, such as processed foods and certain seeds or nuts, can help prevent flare-ups and promote overall gastrointestinal health.

However, dietary changes alone may not be sufficient for managing diverticulitis, especially during acute flare-ups. Medical interventions such as antibiotics, pain management, and, in severe cases, surgery may be necessary to treat complications or recurrent episodes.

Therefore, it's essential for individuals with diverticulitis to work closely with their healthcare providers to develop a comprehensive treatment plan tailored to their specific needs and circumstances.

Furthermore, beyond dietary considerations, adopting a healthy lifestyle can also play a significant role in managing diverticulitis.

Regular exercise, stress management techniques, and smoking cessation can all contribute to better gastrointestinal health and reduce the risk of diverticulitis complications.

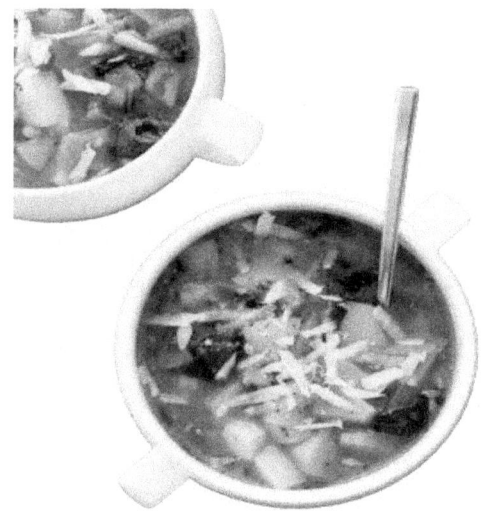

www.ingramcontent.com/pod-product-compliance
Lightning Source LLC
Chambersburg PA
CBHW050259230526
45471CB00005B/1953